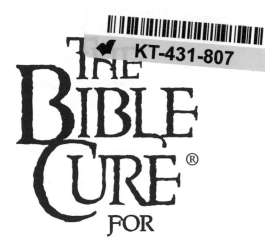

KT-431-807

THE BIBLE CURE® FOR

MEMORY LOSS

DON COLBERT, M.D.

SILOAM

THE BIBLE CURE FOR MEMORY LOSS
by Don Colbert, M.D.
Published by Siloam
Charisma Media/Charisma House Book Group
600 Rinehart Road
Lake Mary, Florida 32746
www.charismahouse.com

Unless otherwise noted, all Scripture quotations are from the Holy Bible, New Living Translation, copyright © 1996. Used by permission of Tyndale House Publishers, Inc., Wheaton, Illinois 60189.

Scripture quotations marked KJV are from the King James Version of the Bible.

Scripture quotations marked NAS are from the New American Standard Bible. Copyright © 1960, 1962, 1963, 1968, 1971, 1972, 1973, 1975, 1977 by the Lockman Foundation. Used by permission. (www.Lockman.org)

Scripture quotations marked NCV are from The Holy Bible, New Century Version. Copyright © 1987, 1988, 1991 by Word Publishing, Dallas, Texas 75039. Used by permission.

Library of Congress Catalog Card Number: 00-193612
International Standard Book Number:
978-0-88419-746-1
E-book ISBN: 978-1-59979-658-1

This publication is translated in Spanish under the title *La cura bíblica para la pérdida de la memoria*, copyright © 2009 by Dr. Don Colbert, published by Casa Creación, a Charisma Media Company. All rights reserved.

This book is not intended to provide medical advice or to take the place of medical advice and treatment from your personal physician. Readers are advised to consult their own doctors or other qualified health professionals regarding the treatment of their medical problems. Neither the publisher nor the author takes any responsibility for any possible consequences from any treatment, action or application of medicine, supplement, herb or preparation to any person reading or following the information in this book. If readers are taking prescription medications, they should consult with their physicians and not take themselves off of medicines to start supplementation without the proper supervision of a physician.

12 13 14 15 16 — 17 16 15 14 13 12
Printed in the United States of America

Don't Accept Memory Loss!

If you are like most people, you probably believe that memory loss is unavoidable, especially as you get older. But did you know that God desires for you to remain just as strong in mind and body as when you were young? Moses' friend Caleb realized God's blessing of a strong mind and body in old age. He said, "I am eighty-five years old today. I am still as strong today as I was in the day Moses sent me; as my strength was then, so my strength is now, for war and for going out and coming in" (Josh. 14:10–11, NAS).

Caleb's mind and body remained strong enough to fight a war, even at eighty-five years of age! What are your expectations for aging? Are you planning to be as sharp when you are eighty-five years old as you are today?

You may be thinking, *That's great for Caleb, but not for me. I'm not even close to being eighty-five years old, and I think I may be experiencing memory loss already!*

It's possible that you have begun to experience a degree of age-associated memory impairment. Later on in this booklet, I invite you to take a detailed test to better determine whether or not you are experiencing memory loss.

Memory Loss and Alzheimer's Disease

Age-related memory loss often starts at about forty-five to fifty years of age. Nearly 15 percent of people experiencing progressive age-related memory loss go on to develop Alzheimer's disease. About one out of every two Americans who are eighty-five and older, and about one out of every ten people who are sixty-five and older, develop Alzheimer's disease. Presently Alzheimer's disease affects about four million people in the United States. These numbers are expected to double and possibly triple in the next fifteen years.

These statistics sound frightening. But memory loss doesn't have to happen to you! Many individuals believe that memory loss is part of growing older. But as Caleb learned, that is simply not true!

A Bold, New Approach

With the help of the practical and faith-inspiring wisdom contained in this Bible Cure booklet, you never have to experience memory loss at all. In addition, it's possible to reverse the process of memory loss if it has already started. Through the power of good nutrition, healthy lifestyle choices, exercise, vitamins and supplements and, most importantly of all, through the power of dynamic faith, you can be empowered to halt the debilitating effects of memory loss.

Memory loss is not your destiny. With God's grace, mental accuracy, power and increasing joy await you at the end of your days!

As you read this book, prepare to win the battle against memory loss. This Bible Cure booklet is filled with practical steps, hope, encouragement and valuable information on how to develop a healthy, empowered lifestyle. In this book, you will

uncover God's divine plan of health
for body, soul and spirit
through modern medicine, good nutrition
and the medicinal power
of Scripture and prayer.

You will also discover life-changing scriptures

throughout this booklet that will strengthen and encourage you.

As you read, apply and trust God's promises, you will also uncover powerful Bible Cure prayers to help you line up your thoughts and feelings with God's plan of divine health for you—a plan that includes living victoriously. In this Bible Cure booklet, you will find powerful insight in the following chapters:

You can confidently take the natural and spiritual steps outlined in this book to combat and defeat memory loss forever.

It is my prayer that these practical suggestions for health, nutrition and fitness will bring wholeness to your life—body, soul and spirit. May they deepen your fellowship with God and strengthen your ability to worship and serve Him.

—DON COLBERT, M.D.

A BIBLE CURE PRAYER
FOR YOU

Mighty God, You are the strength of my body, including my mind. Your Word says that You are no respecter of persons. What You give to one is available to all. You gave Caleb and many others the power of mental accuracy and strength throughout their lives, even in old age. I pray that You help me to receive the gift of a powerful mind through this Bible Cure strategy of divine wisdom, natural methods and supernatural faith. Thank You for the awesome gift of a sharp, keen mind. Fill me with the joy and confidence to praise You right now for victory over memory loss. Amen.

Chapter 1

Wisdom
for the Wise

Memory loss is not your destiny. The Bible says, "The godly will flourish like palm trees and grow strong like the cedars of Lebanon...Even in old age they will still produce fruit; they will remain vital and green. They will declare, 'The Lord is just! He is my rock! There is nothing but goodness in him!'" (Ps. 92:12, 14–15).

Avoiding the pitfalls of aging does not just happen, however. To live a life free from memory loss, you must first gain wisdom. Solomon, the wisest man who ever lived, once said, "My son, give attention to my words; incline your ear to my sayings. Do not let them depart from your sight; keep them in the midst of your heart. For they are life to those who find them, and health to all their whole body" (Prov. 4:20–22, NAS). The health of your whole body includes a healthy, well-functioning mind.

So, let's begin this discussion by carefully investigating memory loss—including any memory loss that you might be experiencing right now. Let's start by determining whether or not you really are experiencing memory loss. Take the Bible Cure test below and tally up your score.

A BIBLE CURE HEALTH TIP

Are You Experiencing Memory Loss?

Take the following test to determine if you are experiencing memory loss.

- ❑ Do you often forget a common word that you use every day and substitute another one in its place?
- ❑ Do you go looking for something, only to forget what it was you were searching for?
- ❑ Do you forget the names of friends?
- ❑ Do you forget appointments?
- ❑ Do you forget the point you were trying to make while talking?
- ❑ Do you misplace keys?

- ❑ Do you find it increasingly difficult to learn new things?
- ❑ Do you find it difficult to add numbers in your head?
- ❑ Do you have difficulty concentrating?
- ❑ Do you depend upon caffeine to be mentally keen?
- ❑ Do you always feel fatigued?
- ❑ Do petty problems frustrate you?
- ❑ Do you frequently repeat yourself?
- ❑ Do you occasionally get lost while driving, even if you have driven there numerous times before?
- ❑ Does your family think that you are more forgetful now compared to before?

If you checked nine or more, you probably have age-associated memory impairment. If you checked twelve or more, you may have early Alzheimer's disease.[1]

Understanding Memory Loss

Now that you've taken the test, you probably have a better indication of where you stand as an individual in regard to memory loss. If you scored high, you don't need to be concerned. After you've gained a better understanding of memory loss, you'll begin to see why.

You don't have to accept the embarrassing symptoms of memory loss as a fact of life. Memory loss can be halted and reversed long before Alzheimer's disease develops. Preventing further decline in memory is much easier than reversing it, so let's gain wisdom about memory loss. What causes memory loss to occur as we age?

If you do nothing to halt or reverse the process, approximately 20 percent of all your brain cells will die over the course of a lifetime. Just as bone mass and muscle mass tend to shrink with age, this cell loss causes the brain mass to shrink as well. Between the ages of twenty and seventy, about 10 percent of brain mass will be lost.

> *Jesus went around doing good and healing all who were oppressed by the Devil, for God was with him.*
> —Acts 10:38

Growing New Brain Cells?

Up until about 1990 most experts believed that it was impossible for the brain to reproduce new cells. Therefore, common wisdom said that nothing could be done about memory loss. It was just a hard fact of growing old.

However, with the development of highly refined tests, experts have discovered that they were very wrong. PET and SPECT scans can map brain activity and measure both the destruction and growth of new brain cells. What these experts discovered was absolutely fascinating— and it completely changed the way we think about memory loss. Thanks to these marvelous advances, today we know that even damaged brains can grow new cells.[2]

Your Brain Cells

Let's take a look at how your brain works. Your thoughts are transmitted through your brain by nerve cells called *neurons*.

Dendrites

If you were able to get inside of your brain, you would see that your brain cells look like an oak tree with thousands of branches, both large and very small. These brain cell branches are called *dendrites*. Dendrites branch out and connect with other brain cells.

The more dendrites your brain has, the better your memory will be. Scientists now know that your incredible brain is able to grow new dendrites, thus forming new thought pathways. This is why an individual who has suffered a stroke and has been paralyzed on one side can learn how to walk again. Even though the stroke killed brain cells, resulting in paralysis, new dendrite branches that were created by the brain went around the dead cells and restored the ability to walk.

Thinking and studying help to form new dendritic connections. So it's critically important to keep mentally active to keep forming new dendritic connections. We'll take a closer look at this in a later chapter.

Synapses

Each brain cell or neuron has many different synapses that enable it to communicate with hundreds of thousands of other nerve cells at lightning speeds. Synapses are the spaces that exist between different neurons or nerve cells. They form a kind of electrical train terminal where messages come in and go out along the nerve cells.

Brain cells not only grow new dendrites and receptors, but they also grow new synapses.

Within the past ten years, scientists have discovered that we can create more message terminal synapses, dendrites and receptors through proper diet, nutritional supplementation, lowering stress and doing physical and mental exercises. If our nerve cells have more synapses and dendrites to transmit brain messages along, then we will have quicker, more accurately functioning brains. We can improve memory and other mental functioning by increasing the connections among our brain cells.

Just as it is possible to improve our physical strength and stamina by applying understanding and wisdom to our lifestyles, so it is also possible to improve our mental functioning in much the same way. It's so simple.

> *But Jesus knew what they were planning. He left that area, and many people followed him. He healed all the sick among them.*
> —Matthew 12:15

The Necessity of Neurotransmitters

We have taken a look at the powerful cells that give us the ability to think and feel. Neurons, or thinking cells, transfer information to each other by using tiny chemicals called neurotransmitters. Neurotransmitters are stored in bags called *vesicles* inside the nerve cells and are released as needed.

Neurotransmitters are chemicals that are released in the brain when we think. They are released across the synapses and unite to receiver cells (receptor sites) on other nerve cells. The incredible neurotransmitters form the very essence of our intelligence, memory and mood. Different neurotransmitters also have specific functions.

Approximately fifty different varieties of these incredible chemicals have been identified in the brain. Some of the most important neurotransmitters include acetylcholine,

> *But he was wounded and crushed for our sins. He was beaten that we might have peace. He was whipped, and we were healed!*
> —ISAIAH 53:5

norepinephrine, dopamine, serotonin and GABA. Which type of neurotransmitters that your neurons make and release is actually dependent upon what you eat. Let's take a closer look at these brain chemicals.

Acetylcholine

The most important neurotransmitter for memory and thought is acetylcholine. If you have been experiencing difficulty concentrating, it may well be because your body lacks acetylcholine. Acetylcholine is made from choline, which is found in egg yolks. Your brain has more of this neuro-transmitter than any of the other types.

Norepinephrine

Norepinephrine helps to transfer short-term memories to long-term storage. Norepinephrine also helps to elevate your mood. Your body is able to make its own norepinephrine from two important amino acids (L-tyrosine and L-phenylalanine).

Serotonin

Serotonin gives you a feeling of well-being and helps you sleep. You can increase the amount of serotonin in your body by eating tryptophan, which is an amino acid found in turkey meat. Other sources of tryptophan include milk, cheese, legumes, cashews, dates, figs, bananas and spinach.

Dopamine

Dopamine affects your memory, mood and sex drive. If the levels of dopamine in your body become too low, you could end up with Parkinson's disease. Dopamine helps the body to move freely rather than rigidly as the bodies of Parkinson's patients tend to do.

GABA

GABA is a calming neurotransmitter and is

critically important for sleep and relaxation. Without GABA, our minds would be overstimulated, and we would eventually become exhausted.

Are You Left-Brained or Right-Brained?

Your brain is divided into two halves, or two hemispheres, called the right and left. You usually use one side of your brain much more than the other side. Therefore, one side of your brain is usually much more developed than the other side. An extremely small percentage of individuals actually use both sides of their brains equally—this is extremely rare. These people are called ambidextrous.

Right-brained people

Do you like to draw and paint? Are you good at making crafts? If so, you may be right-brained.

If you are right-brained, you may be an artist or a musician. You may even be an architect or an engineer. The right side of the brain is mainly involved with creativity, music, spatial organization, recognition of faces and mathematics.

More men than women tend to be right-brained.

Left-brained people

Are you fluent in many languages? Do you enjoy crossword puzzles and word games? Do you love poetry and discussing many different topics, great and small? Are you an excellent organizer or a good bookkeeper? If so, you may be left-brained.

The left side of the brain is primarily involved with language and analytical processes. More women than men tend to be left-brained.

Short-Term
and Long-Term Memory

Just as your family room is the center of activity for your family—or is it your kitchen?—your brain has a memory-central also. The limbic system of the brain is its main memory center, and it is here that both short-term and long-term memories are processed.

Memories travel through your brain like electrical charges through this system. The limbic system is composed of five main divisions. They are the:

- Hippocampus
- Amygdala
- Hypothalamus

- Thalamus
- Pituitary

Just as an efficient secretary stores important information in organized files and cabinets, your brain does the same. After your memories are processed and sorted under long-term, short-term and emotional memories, they are sent to storage facilities. The hippocampus stores your short-term and long-term memories. Then it transfers most of the long-term memories to the neocortex, which is a part of the large gray matter of the brain. The amygdala of the limbic system processes emotional memories. The more emotional a thought is, the more likely it is to be stored long term in the amygdala.

The cerebrum actually looks like two halves of a walnut with grooves and fissures. The cerebrum is covered by a one- to two-millimeter coating called the neocortex, or "thinking brain."

> *And the Lord's healing power was strongly with Jesus.*
> —Luke 5:17

What's the difference between short-term and long-term memory? That's easy. Think about your first-grade teacher. What was her name? You

12

probably remember, don't you? What about the children in your first-grade class? You may be able to name them all, supplying both their first and last names. OK, now recite the last phone number you looked up in the yellow pages. Can you remember? Probably not! Do you know why? The phone number was stored in your short-term memory, and your first-grade information was stored in your long-term memory.

Your mind knew that you didn't need to store the phone number information forever, so it flushed it out immediately after you used it.

A Senior Moment

The memory loss associated with aging is called *age-associated memory impairment*, but many seniors prefer to say they are simply having a "senior moment." But be careful not to confuse terms. *Dementia*, although once called senility, is memory impairment on a much greater scale.

The Devastation of Dementia

Common signs of dementia include the following:

- **Language difficulties,** such as forgetting normal words or the phrasing of words in such a way that speech is not understood.

- **Confusion of time and place.** Individuals with dementia may get lost in their homes, may forget what year or month it is and may not recognize loved ones whom they've known for years.

- **Difficulty with familiar tasks.** Dementia sufferers may walk out of a store without paying.

- **Lack of judgment.** Dementia patients may put their clothes on backwards or inside out, or may go swimming and forget to wear their swimming suits.

Alzheimer's Disease

In patients with Alzheimer's disease, the hippocampus is one of the first areas of the brain to be damaged. Since short-term memories are stored in the hippocampus, Alzheimer's patients lose their short-term memories first. They lose their long-term memories, which are mainly stored in the neocortex, much later.

Causes of Dementia

More than sixty diseases are capable of causing dementia. However, Alzheimer's disease is responsible for more dementia than all other causes combined.

What Happens During Alzheimer's?

Patients with Alzheimer's disease suffer from some major changes in their brain tissue.

First, brain cells develop abnormal fibers called *neurofibrillary tangles*. These tangles interfere with the function of the brain cells and eventually kill them.

In addition, the brain cells accumulate senile plaques, which are dead cellular material that accumulate around a protein (called amyloid).

The brain of an Alzheimer's patient is also extremely deficient in the most important neurotransmitter acetylcholine.

Researchers have discovered that Alzheimer's disease is linked to a certain gene, apolipoprotein E. If an individual carries two apolipoprotein E-4 genes, he or she may have more than 90 percent chance of developing Alzheimer's by the age of eighty.

Don't Fear

By now you must realize what a complex, wonderful creation your brain is. No computer has ever been made or will ever be made to rival it. If you've seen yourself or your loved ones in this information on memory loss, please don't let your heart become fearful. This booklet is written to provide you with the power to reverse the symptoms and stop the progression of memory loss in its tracks.

The Bible says, "Let not your heart be troubled, neither let it be afraid" (John 14:27, KJV). There is no disease, no problem and no symptom that cannot be conquered through faith, God's powerful Word and His divine wisdom.

> *So Jesus healed great numbers of sick people who had many different kinds of diseases.*
> —MARK 1:34

So, as you discover powerful biblical and natural wisdom throughout the following pages of this booklet to halt and reverse memory loss, get ready to win!

A BIBLE CURE PRAYER
FOR YOU

Lord Jesus, I choose to look to You right now for all of my answers, even for any deep concerns I have about memory loss. I place my fears before You, and I ask You to teach me Your own wisdom and understanding about memory loss. Build up my faith, and help me see You as the powerful answer to all of my problems. Amen.

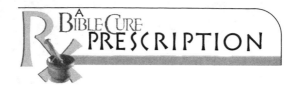

Do you feel that you or a loved one are experiencing memory loss?

_____

List any person or persons whom you feel may have symptoms of dementia or Alzheimer's disease.

_____

_____

Write a prayer committing that person or persons to God's care. Thank God for revealing this knowledge about preventing memory loss.

_____

_____

_____

_____

_____

Chapter 2

Food for Thought

Some people scoff at the notion that what they eat can actually impact their mental functioning. But a lack of knowledge can have disastrous consequences. God spoke of this matter in the Bible when He said, "My people are destroyed for lack of knowledge" (Hos. 4:6, NAS).

Diet and nutrition have a direct and powerful impact upon memory loss and are key factors in your ability to halt and reverse any symptoms that you may be experiencing.

Getting wise counsel so you can become better informed about diet and memory loss is vital. Are you ready to become a little wiser? The Word of God says, "A wise man will hear and increase in learning, and a man of understanding will acquire wise counsel" (Prov. 1:5, NAS).

Years ago, Hippocrates, the father of medicine,

surmised that certain foods were good for the brain. He said that food that is good for the heart is likely to be good for the brain as well. He had no evidence to make his statement, just the wisdom gained from years of study and observation about how the human body works. Today we know that Hippocrates was absolutely right. Let's take a look.

We're All Fat Heads

Have you ever been called a fat head? If so, the person who called you that was more correct than he or she probably ever imagined. Let me explain.

The brain is actually made up of fat. Believe it or not, that makes it the body's fattiest organ. The brain is actually made

> *O Lord, you alone can heal me; you alone can save.*
> —Jeremiah 17:14

from about 60 percent of fatty substances called lipids. Therefore, it's very important that we eat the proper kinds of fat to nourish the brain's cells.

Diet for a Healthy Brain

Every brain cell is covered by a cell membrane composed of two layers of fats called phospholipids. Your brain cell membranes must be flexible and pliable to communicate easily and accurately with other cells in the brain.

When you eat bad fats, such as saturated and hydrogenated fats, the brain cell membranes may become stiff and rigid.

The Dangers of Hydrogenated Fats

If you looked at the brain's communicator chemicals, the neurotransmitters, under a microscope, the first thing you would notice is that each one has a unique shape all its own.

Each of these differently shaped neurotransmitters must fit into the "receivers," or the receptors, of the nerve cell. This process normally works quite easily and well. But if the membranes have been made hard and rigid by bad fats, then the receptors will also become rigid. When this happens, the receptor is unable to alter its shape to allow the neurotransmitter to bind or act like a key unlocking a lock. Communication between brain cells is short-circuited, and memory loss occurs.

The worse fats for the brain are hydrogenated fats, also known as trans fatty acids. You can find hydrogenated fats in the following products:

- Margarine
- Most peanut butters
- Salad dressing
- Shortening

These fats also cause the cell membranes to thicken and harden and lose their ability to allow enough nutrients to come into the cells. When this occurs, wastes are also prevented from leaving the cells. Both of these factors increase memory loss symptoms.

Um, Uh, Well . . .
What Saturated Fats Can Do

How many of us haven't found ourselves standing in front of someone painfully trying to pull up vital information that we know, only to draw a blank?

Perhaps you've been eating too much saturated fat and your receptors have become hard and rigid.

Saturated fats have much the same effect as hydrogenated fats upon memory loss. Heavy loads of saturated fats are found in the following foods:

- Hamburgers
- French fries
- Butter
- Fried foods
- Baked goods
- Red meat

If these foods are the mainstay of your diet, you could be in trouble. If you have noticed some memory loss symptoms, you may have plenty of the neurotransmitters in your brain to carry information. But if your cell membranes have become rigid, that information cannot make the necessary connections, causing your memory to lose its edge.

But if you've watched the saturated and hydrogenated fats and have eaten plenty of Omega-3 fat, then your cell membrane receptors will be softer and more pliable. They will easily accept neurotransmitters. Now you're ready to become a contestant on *Who Wants to Be a Millionaire?* or *Jeopardy!*

The Miracle of Omega-3 Fats

Foods containing Omega-3 fats are brain enhancers. So, for a keen mind, load up your plate often with Omega-3 choices. Some of these are as follows:

- Fish oils
- Salmon
- Mackerel
- Sardines
- Herring
- Tuna
- Flaxseed oil

Omega-3s are the most fluid fats and thus help to keep brain cell membranes soft and pliable. If only 50 percent of your receptor sites are soft and pliable, then you may be getting only 50 percent of the messages your neurotransmitters are sending. This may be the reason why so many people lack razor-sharp minds—perhaps only half of their brain messages are able to get through.

Flaxseed oil is also a highly concentrated form of Omega-3 fat. Try to take 1–2 tablespoons daily.

More Brainpower Through Fish and DHA

Fish is a brainpower food. If you enjoy eating fish, you're in very good company. It was one of the most common foods eaten in the Bible. Jesus miraculously multiplied it to feed the

> *He personally carried away our sins in his own body on the cross so we can be dead to sin and live for what is right. You have been healed by his wounds!*
> —1 PETER 2:24

multitudes, and He prepared it several times for His disciples. In fact, quite a few of the disciples were fishermen. Learn to enjoy eating fish several times a week.

One form of fish's Omega-3 fatty acid is called

DHA. It has been discovered that the more DHA a food contains, the higher the level of serotonin. Serotonin is a neurotransmitter that actually causes you to feel a greater sense of well-being. Prozac is also able to raise the serotonin in the brain. But it is much safer to eat foods containing DHA.

Your body cannot make sufficient amounts of DHA to supply your brain's needs. Therefore it is important that you get DHA in your diet on a daily basis. DHA is found in the following types of fish:

- Mackerel
- Sardines
- Herring
- Salmon
- Tuna
- Whitefish

DHA helps to create flexible brain structures. Patients diagnosed with Alzheimer's disease are twice as likely to have low levels of DHA in their blood. In addition, normal individuals who tested with low blood levels of DHA had a two-thirds greater risk of developing Alzheimer's disease in the following ten years.

Fish oil or Omega-3 fatty acids also prevent a buildup of substances, called leukotrienes and cytokines, that produce inflammation. The inflammation caused by these agents can also interfere with memory and can injure blood vessels.

Avoid Excessive Amounts of
Polyunsaturated Fats

Polyunsaturated fats, which include safflower oil, sunflower oil, corn oil and soybean oil, are also damaging to the brain. Another word for polyunsaturated fats is Omega-6 fatty acids. These fats oxidize much faster than other forms of fat and create free radicals that can damage the brain.

Eating too much polyunsaturated fat can destroy DHA. It is critically important to lower our intake of these potentially dangerous fats.

Magnificent Monounsaturated Fats

Monounsaturated fats are very good fats that help prevent bad cholesterol (LDL cholesterol, or low-density lipoprotein) from oxidizing. They can be found in the following foods:

- Extra-virgin olive oil
- Canola oil
- Almonds
- Macadamia nut oil
- Flaxseed oil
- Avocados

If you want to improve your memory, stop using regular salad dressings. Instead, switch to extra-virgin olive oil or flaxseed oil with vinegar.

Changing the types of fats and oils you use is

not the only dietary requirement for developing and maintaining a keenly functioning mind. Sugar is another key factor to consider.

Sweet Memories

Glucose, or sugar, is the brain's exclusive source of fuel. Therefore, getting enough is important. However, most Americans take in way too much sugar. The average individual consumes about 150 pounds of sugar per year.

Too much sugar will also contribute toward lower mental functioning. Let me explain why.

Insulin and Blood Sugar

Too much sugar in your blood will cause your pancreas to release insulin to lower the sugar level in your blood.

Insulin is a hormone produced by your pancreas that regulates the amount of sugar in your blood. The body converts the food you eat into a form of sugar—glucose—and distributes it to the cells of the body through the bloodstream.

Each cell is a self-contained structure with a delicate environment. The cell membranes will not allow certain substances to enter without a "key" or "gatekeeper" to allow entrance into the cell. Insulin is the body's key that allows glucose to leave the bloodstream and enter a cell.

Under normal circumstances, the pancreas efficiently manages the level of sugar in our blood day after day, year after year without incident. Frankly, most people rarely think about their pancreas unless a problem develops.

High levels of sugar in your blood cause high levels of insulin to be released into your bloodstream. Maintaining these high levels for too long by regularly eating too much sugar and too many processed carbohydrates will cause your body to produce a regular oversupply of insulin. When this happens, your body can begin to become insulin resistant.

Insulin resistance means that the insulin receptors on the body's cells—the gatekeepers or keys—stop functioning properly. This is usually an early stage of adult-onset diabetes. Too much sugar may cause your body's cells to begin refusing to allow sugar or glucose into the cells at all.

Remember that glucose is the brain's exclusive source of fuel. If you are becoming insulin resistant, in other words, if your insulin is not working effectively to allow the sugar into your cells, then the brain cells may not get enough glucose.

What happens when your car doesn't have enough fuel to run? That's easy—it can't run. Well, since your brain uses sugar or glucose as fuel, if your cells stop receiving it, your brain stops getting it. The result is memory loss.

Therefore, it's vitally important that you do not overload your body with sugar and carbohydrates that will elevate your insulin to unsafe levels. Eating sugary foods all the time is very dangerous, and it can eventually result in memory loss. However, many carbohydrates increase blood sugar levels in your body in much the same way.

Culprit Carbs

The following Bible Cure HealthFact contains a glycemic index to help you determine how much glucose your diet may be producing. The amount of fiber in your food, the amount of fat and proteins, in addition to how much sugar is in the carbohydrates, all determine the glycemic index score of what you eat.

Glycemic Index of Foods

EXTREMELY HIGH (GREATER THAN 100)

Corn flakes

Millet

Potato, baked, instant

Honey

Rice, instant, puffed

Bread, French

Carrots, cooked

GLYCEMIC STANDARD = 100 PERCENT

Bread, white

HIGH (80–100)

Bread, rye, wheat,
whole meal

Grape Nuts

Muesli

Crispbread

Corn, sweet

Potato, broiled, mashed

Apricots

Banana

Mango

Pastry

Crackers

Shredded wheat

Tortilla, corn

Rice, brown, white

Raisins

Papaya

Candy bars

Cookies

Ice cream, low fat

Corn chips

MODERATELY HIGH (60–80)

Buckwheat

Bread, rye, pumpernickel

Macaroni, white

Yams

Green peas

All Bran

Bulgur

Spaghetti, white, brown

Sweet potatoes

Green peas (frozen)

Baked beans (canned)   Kidney beans (canned)
Fruit cocktail   Grapefruit juice
Orange juice   Pineapple juice
Pears (canned)   Grapes
Oatmeal cookies   Potato chips
Sponge cake

Moderate (40–60)

White beans   Tomato soup
Green peas, dried   Lima beans
Butter beans   Chickpeas (garbanzo)
Kidney beans   Black-eyed peas
Black beans   Apple juice
Orange   Apple
Pears   Milk
Yogurt

Low (less than 40)

Barley   Soybeans
Red lentils   Plums
Peaches   Peanuts
Fructose

HEALTHFACT HEALTHFACT HEALTHFACT HEALTHFACT HEALTHFACT HEALTHFACT HEALTHFACT

Free Radicals and Memory Loss

Insulin resistance is not the only way in which eating too much sugar produces memory loss. Another culprit is called AGEs, or advanced glycosylation end products.

AGEs are produced when the sugar (or glucose) in your blood reacts with proteins that are also in your blood. This reaction creates a protein substance that builds up in your cells in much the same way that plaque builds up on your teeth after a day of not brushing. This buildup is called AGEs.

The higher the sugar levels in your diet, the more AGEs are created in your bloodstream. If you get enough of this sugar/protein buildup, you will actually age faster! It also creates brain-damaging free radicals that increase memory loss.

Fighting Free
Radicals With Antioxidants

Antioxidants help defend the brain from free-radical damage. (We will take an in-depth look at antioxidants and free radicals in the next chapter.) Many antioxidants are found naturally in fruits and vegetables. Those with the deepest color usually contain the highest amounts of antioxidants. Listed below are some fruits and vegetables in which you can find the highest level of antioxidants.

- Prunes
- Garlic
- Cranberries
- Strawberries
- Spinach
- Raspberries

Eating these fruits and vegetables will help save your brain from free-radical destruction. Let's look at some other powerful sources as well.

Grape juice has four times more antioxidant capacity than other juices, including grapefruit juice, tomato juice and orange juice. However, do not drink too much since it also contains sugar.

Black tea and green tea are very high in anti-oxidant potency. However, instant teas, herbal teas and bottled teas have little or no anti-oxidant activity.

> But for you who fear my name, the Sun of Righteousness will rise with healing in his wings. And you will go free, leaping with joy like calves let out to pasture.
> —MALACHI 4:2

Red wine is also full of antioxidants, but teas and red grape juice can give you as much protection as red wine, and without the alcohol. Therefore, I definitely prefer these beverages to red wine.

Blood Sugar Too Low?

Just as high blood sugar can impact mental functioning, low blood sugar can also have an effect. If brain cells do not have enough glucose, the mitochondria, which are the energy-producing portions of the brain cells, cannot produce enough energy. This can result in memory problems and mood swings. Such symptoms are commonly experienced by people with hypoglycemia who become irritable, foggy-headed or agitated when they miss a meal.

Your brain needs to have an adequate, consistent and steady supply of glucose to function at peak performance. This is why your body works hard to maintain a fairly constant level of glucose in the blood in

> *But the crowds found out where he was going, and they followed him. And he welcomed them, teaching them about the Kingdom of God and curing those who were ill.*
> —LUKE 9:11

order to service the brain. But you can help your body keep your glucose levels fairly constant by eating every three to four hours.

Don't skip meals! When you skip meals, your blood sugar drops lower and your brain functioning is affected. Keeping a forty-thirty-thirty supplement bar nearby for midmorning and midafternoon munchies will help to keep your blood sugar levels constant. The following HealthTip gives some additional eating tips that will help you to maintain a razor-sharp mind.[1]

Eating Tips

It's best to eat the protein portion of your meal first since this stimulates glucagon, which depresses insulin secretion and releases carbohydrates stored in your liver and muscles, helping to prevent low blood sugar.

- Eat slowly and chew each bite at least twenty to thirty times.

- Never eat when you are upset, angry or bickering. Eating should be a time of relaxation and should never be hurried since hydrochloric acid will be suppressed and your food will not be able to be digested well.

- Limit your starches to only one serving per meal. In other words, don't eat bread, pasta, potatoes, corn and different starches together at one meal. This elevates insulin levels. If you do go back for seconds, choose fruits, vegetables and salads, but not starches.

- If you are craving a dessert, simply eliminate the starch or the bread, pasta, potatoes and corn and have a small dessert. However, be sure to have your protein and fat since this will balance out the sugar in the dessert. But don't make desserts a regular habit. Save them for special occasions such as birthdays, holidays and anniversaries.

- Be sure that your diet has plenty of fiber. Fiber actually slows down the digestion and absorption of carbohydrates.

- Avoid alcoholic beverages, not only because alcohol is toxic to our bodies, but also because it triggers a tremendous insulin release and promotes storage of fat.

Conclusion

Sometimes applying a little wisdom and understanding can have powerful results. If you are experiencing memory loss, it may be that you simply need to make a few minor adjustments in what and when you eat.

If you find yourself reaching for breads and cakes to fill an emotional void in your life, consider this: Jesus Christ is the Bread of Life.

Seeking His wisdom, help and strength will completely transform your life—even the way you eat and think. His power to save knows no limits. When you are tempted to eat the wrong things, remember His promise to you: "I am the bread of life. No one who comes to me will ever be hungry again. Those who believe in me will never thirst" (John 6:35).

A BIBLE CURE PRAYER
FOR YOU

Dear Lord, I give You all my unhealthy eating habits that may be contributing to my memory loss. Please give me the strength I need to avoid sugary foods, breads, processed foods and bad fats. Give me a divine grace to desire what is good for my body and to stay determined to make healthy choices even when I am tempted. Thank You for Your great love for me, and thank You that You are working in my life to free me from the disabling effects of memory loss. In Jesus' name, amen.

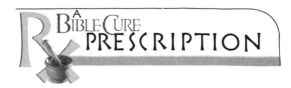

A BIBLE CURE PRESCRIPTION

Write down some ways that you can begin to introduce good fats into your diet.

_____

_____

_____

_____

List poor eating habits you currently have and why they may be adding to memory loss.

_____

_____

_____

Write a prayer asking God to help you overcome any poor eating habits you may have.

_____

_____

_____

_____

Chapter 3

Supplements
for Brainpower

God promises special, supernatural protection
and care to those who seek His help. If you
heed sound, biblical wisdom regarding your
mind and body, you can enjoy God's special protection. The Bible says, "If you make the LORD
your refuge, if you make the Most High your
shelter, no evil will conquer you; no plague will
come near your dwelling" (Ps. 91:9–10).

Too many people believe that God will protect
and help them with crisis-sized problems such as
cancer or a heart attack. Others believe God will
help them with minor issues in life, but not major
ones. Both of these positions are wrong. God
cares deeply about you, and He is deeply concerned about every issue in your life—large and
small. No concern is too big or too little to miss
His care.

Perhaps you've never even considered asking God for help with memory loss, especially if you've seen it as a minor inconvenience of growing old. But God's grace and protection extend to every area of your life, even memory loss. So let's take a look at some important factors involved in memory loss that you may have never considered.

If you're like many of us, you probably feel that the food you eat provides you with all the nutrients you need to maintain a healthy functioning mind and body. But modern farming methods that strip soil of vital nutrients, coupled with today's diet of processed foods, make it nearly impossible to nourish our bodies adequately with food alone. Sound nutritional wisdom demands that we support our daily meals with supplements. When it comes to combating memory loss, supplementation is essential! Let's take an in-depth look at why this is so.

Oxygen and Your Brain

Your brain needs a great deal of oxygen to function properly. As a matter of fact, it requires more oxygen than any other organ in the body—about 25 percent of all the blood pumped by the heart is used by the brain.

Because of the enormous amount of oxygen the brain requires, it also generates more free radicals than any other tissue in the body. Free radicals are a kind of molecular shrapnel.

To understand free radicals, consider the process of oxidation. Burn wood in a fireplace, and smoke is a by-product. Likewise, when you metabolize food into energy, oxygen oxidizes (or burns) the food to produce energy. This process does not create smoke, but it does produce dangerous by-products known as free radicals. These are molecules with unpaired electrons that cause damage to other cells.

> *If you will listen carefully to the voice of the LORD your God and do what is right in his sight, obeying his commands and laws, then I will not make you suffer the diseases I sent on the Egyptians; for I am the LORD who heals you.*
> —EXODUS 15:26

Free radicals can create cellular havoc in your brain, damaging many of the brain's functions we've looked at thus far. One of the primary reasons is that the brain is a fatty organ, as we have already seen. Fat is a major target for free radicals. When the fat in the brain cell membranes becomes oxidized, it can eventually lead to conditions such as Alzheimer's and Parkinson's disease.

Oxidized fat becomes rancid in the cell membranes, which drastically changes the way they function. Receptors and neurotransmitters are tremendously altered, as is the way in which glucose is transported and received in the brain. Free radicals can also cripple the brain's ability to produce energy as well.

Your Busy Brain That Never Sleeps

Another reason that the brain forms large amounts of free radicals is because the brain never stops working. Brain cells need a constant supply of both blood and oxygen. Therefore, significant amounts of free radicals are produced continually.

In addition, when brain cell membranes become rancid, cells can no longer move calcium out and glucose into the cells. This means that calcium levels can rise to toxic levels, which increases free-radical damage even more. This can actually lead to the death of brain cells.

A Patriot Missile Defense System

Like molecular Patriot missiles, antioxidants stop free radicals in their tracts before they can damage your body. But the brain appears to have a somewhat deficient natural supply of these defense weapons compared to the rest of the body, according to Dr. James Joseph, chief of neuroscience at the U.S. Department of Agriculture, Human Nutrition Research Center on Aging at Tufts University.[1] This is why taking the right supplements is vital to arresting and reversing memory loss.

Dr. Lester Packer, professor of molecular and cell biology at the University of California at Berkeley, believes that the

> *A man shall be commended according to his wisdom.*
> —PROVERBS 12:8, KJV

body's best defense against free radicals is a network of antioxidants. Dr. Packer sees five extraordinary antioxidants as making up this network:[2]

- Vitamin E
- Vitamin C
- Coenzyme Q_{10}
- Lipoic acid
- Glutathione

These antioxidants join together to form an impenetrable shield against free-radical attacks. When one antioxidant fails to neutralize a free-radical hit, another launches to back it up.

Vitamin C or coenzyme Q_{10} can donate electrons to revive a failed vitamin E hit. And lipoic acid can resuscitate all the other antioxidants in addition to itself.

Defending Against Diseases

Antioxidants certainly are powerful! Not only do they wage cellular warfare with free radicals, but they also protect your genes from triggering genetic diseases. You see, free radicals are known to activate disease-related genes in the nucleus of the cell. But with adequate amounts of antioxidants in your bloodstream, antioxidants can help to prevent neurodegenerative diseases such as Parkinson's disease and Alzheimer's disease.

A Closer Look at the
Patriot Missile Defense Team

The brain-protecting antioxidant defense team— – vitamin E, vitamin C, glutathione, coenzyme Q_{10} and lipoic acid—can be taken as daily supplements. If you've been experiencing some symptoms of memory loss, beginning this supplementation regimen may give you immediate relief. Let's take a closer look.

Vitamin E

Vitamin E protects the fat in cell membranes from turning rancid. In April 1997, the *New England Journal of Medicine* reported that the debilitating symptoms of Alzheimer's disease were reduced in half of Alzheimer's patients who took 1000 IUs of vitamin E daily.[3]

Some experts say that about 30 percent of Americans have a vitamin E deficiency. In addition, all developed countries are slightly deficient in vitamin E.[4]

> *Yes, your healing will come quickly.*
> —Isaiah 58:8

Take 400 IUs of natural vitamin E daily for antioxidant protection. Dosages of 800 IUs or more may thin the blood. Therefore, check with your physician before taking more than 400 IUs.

Vitamin C

The antioxidant vitamin C actually donates electrons to help regenerate vitamin E. The brain also uses vitamin C to make the neurotransmitters dopamine and adrenaline. Vitamin C also increases levels of glutathione, which is one of the most important antioxidants in the body.

Take 500 milligrams of vitamin C two to three times a day.

Coenzyme Q_{10}

Coenzyme Q_{10} is an extremely important brain-enhancing antioxidant because it protects the fats in the brain from turning rancid. This free-radical damage, called lipid peroxidation, can kill brain cells.

Coenzyme Q_{10} also helps to recycle vitamin E, and it helps to produce energy in the brain. Like a Patriot missile, coenzyme Q_{10} quenches free radicals before they damage nerve cell membranes. Patients with Parkinson's disease tend to have very low levels of coenzyme Q_{10} in their bloodstreams.

Take at least 30 milligrams of coenzyme Q_{10} a day. If you smoke, if you're experiencing memory loss or if you have heart disease, take at least 100–200 milligrams of coenzyme Q_{10} daily.

Lipoic acid

Lipoic acid is the most powerful of all the other antioxidants. It easily penetrates the blood brain barrier in the fatty and water-soluble portions of cells. It is also the only antioxidant that can recycle itself.

Lipoic acid not only neutralizes free radicals, but it also increases the efficiency of mitochondria. This powerful defender helps to control insulin and blood sugar by preventing AGEs, which we already know tend to accelerate aging.

Take at least 100 milligrams of lipoic acid daily, 50 milligrams in the morning and 50 milligrams in the afternoon. If you are diabetic, you may increase that dosage to 600–900 milligrams per day.

Glutathione

The fifth powerful antioxidant needed daily by the brain is glutathione. But it's not easy to increase levels of this powerful antioxidant with food or supplements. Taking lipoic acid will actually raise your glutathione levels, and it will help your body to recycle the glutathione that it already has.

You may choose to take glutathione supplements. Take 250 milligrams twice per day.

Supplements of N-acetyl-cysteine can also raise your glutathione.

> *Dear friend,*
> *I am praying that*
> *all is well with you*
> *and that your body*
> *is as healthy as I*
> *know your soul is.*
> —3 JOHN 2

If you choose this alternative, then take 500 milligrams twice a day.

Whey protein, L-glutamine and broccoli are also good sources of glutathione.

Ginkgo biloba

Ginkgo biloba is one of the most important supplements for rejuvenating memory. This powerful supplement enhances the flow of blood and oxygen to the brain, and it is a powerful antioxidant.

A 1997 double-blind study published by the *Journal of the American Medical Association* shows that ginkgo peps up mental ability.[5] Ginkgo biloba is an effective treatment in many cases of age-related memory impairment, absentmindedness and problems with concentration. It has even improved some milder cases of Alzheimer's disease.[6]

A double-blind study showed that a single 600-milligram dose of ginkgo caused a significant improvement in short-term memory within one hour in patients who had memory loss.[7]

Ginkgo helps to improve short-term memory, and it speeds up reaction times. It will help you to store and retrieve recently learned information such as phone numbers and lists of words more quickly and accurately.

If you have a mild degree of memory loss, I recommend approximately 120 milligrams one to two times a day. If you are experiencing a significant degree of memory loss or the initial stages of

Alzheimer's disease, I recommend taking 120 milligrams two to three times per day.

Phosphatidyl serine

Phosphatidyl serine (PS) is simply a form of fat that is present in all cell membranes. As I've already mentioned, the fatty brain is composed of about 60 percent of fatlike substances called phospholipids.

Phospholipids are more abundant in the brain than in any other organ in the body. PS also has no trouble crossing the blood brain barrier where it helps neurons to better communicate with one another. It does this by raising the levels of neurotransmitters, especially dopamine and acetylcholine.

In addition, PS helps to speed up nerve impulses, and it helps to prevent dendrite connections from being destroyed by aging.

Researcher Thomas H. Crook III, Ph.D., of the National Institute of Mental Health says phosphatidyl serine has a powerful effect on memory. Studies done in 1991 on 149 patients with age-related memory impairment showed remarkable results. For twelve weeks half of the study group patients took 100 milligrams of PS three times a day, and the other half took a placebo (sugar pill).

The group taking PS turned the clock back by twelve years in memory decline in specific tests of memory performance. This included tests for misplaced objects, written material and for recall of phone numbers. The test subjects were also better able to concentrate while talking, reading and performing other tasks.

Crook believes that PS can roll back the clock on memory loss for all age-associated memory impairment. However, PS has not been as effective in treating advanced Alzheimer's disease.[8]

If you have begun to notice any degree of memory loss, it's important to begin taking PS right away to prevent Alzheimer's. Some studies show that PS reduces cortisol, which is a substance that can cause the death of brain cells.[9]

PS supplements are made from soybeans and can be found at most health food stores. Since they tend to be expensive, I recommend taking 100 milligrams three times a day at mealtimes for one month. Following that first month, reduce the dosage to 100 milligrams per day.

Acetyl L-carnitine

Carnitine is a vitamin-like substance that's used for conditions such as congestive heart failure and angina. Acetyl L-carnitine (ALC) is a special form of carnitine that aids mental functioning.

ALC increases energy across the brain's mito-chondrial membrane, and it improves communi-cation between the brain's two hemispheres. ALC appears to be much more effective for patients with early age-associated memory impairment.

If you are experiencing mild memory impair-ment, take 500 milligrams of ALC daily. If you are experiencing moderate to severe memory impair-ment, take 500 milligrams three times a day.

DMAE

DMAE, otherwise known as dimethylamine ethanol, helps the body to produce a major thought and memory neurotransmitter called acetylcholine. DMAE not only helps to improve short-term memory, but it also helps improve concentration. If you have bipolar disorder or epilepsy, do not take DMAE.

I recommend 50–100 milligrams of DMAE two to three times a day in the morning and at noon (since it causes insomnia in some people).

Choline

Choline is an amino acid, which is the raw material necessary for the synthesis of acetyl-choline. This most abundant neurotransmitter in the brain is concentrated in the hippocampus, the brain's memory center. If you do not have enough acetylcholine in your brain, you will have memory problems and a difficult time concentrating.

Choline is also an important component in the fatty membranes of brain cells. Your body is not able to make enough acetylcholine, so it depends upon you to eat food that will help it get this vital neurotransmitter.

One of the richest sources of choline is egg yolks. However, many Americans no longer eat eggs due to the high cholesterol found in them. A recent study by Harvard researchers concluded that an egg a day is not likely to increase the risk of heart disease and strokes.[10] Other foods high in choline include fish, peanuts, meat, cheese, cabbage and broccoli.

Taking lecithin capsules is an excellent way to be sure your body is getting all the choline it needs for a healthy functioning brain. Take at least 500 milligrams a day of choline, which may be obtained with lecithin capsules or granules.

Huperzine A

Huperzine A is actually a plant extract derived from Chinese club moss. It is believed that Huperzine A blocks the enzyme that destroys the neurotransmitter acetylcholine. Levels of acetylcholine tend to be very low in Alzheimer's patients. Therefore Huperzine A acts very similarly to drugs used to treat Alzheimer's disease.

Huperzine A can be found in health food stores and is extremely safe compared to medications used for Alzheimer's. Huperzine appears to be most effective in individuals with advanced cases of Alzheimer's. It may not be as beneficial to those with mild to moderate memory loss.

Take 100 micrograms of Huperzine A a day, and increase it to 200 micrograms twice a day if needed.

Ginseng

Ginseng is a stress-busting supplement that helps your body handle the devastating effects of stress. It does this by protecting your body from producing too much cortisol. Excess cortisol damages brain cells, thus causing memory loss.

Three different herbs are all given the name ginseng, so it's important to know what you're buying. Asian, or Korean ginseng, is also known as Panax ginseng. In addition, American and Siberian ginseng varieties exist.

Ginseng must be grown for approximately five years before it's harvested. Therefore, it usually commands a very high price. However, the quality of ginseng can vary dramatically.

Siberian ginseng is generally considered the best for memory loss. Take 300–400 milligrams of Siberian ginseng extract two to three times a day. Take it for three weeks, followed by a one-week rest period.

Green tea

Green tea contains antioxidants called polyphenols. These powerful substances increase antioxidant activity in the blood up to 50 percent. Green tea is also rich in flavonoids, which can help prevent blood clots and may reduce the incidence of mini-strokes, which also cause memory loss. Many different kinds of flavonoids exist, including bioflavonoids, pine bark extract and grape seed extract.

To a lesser extent, black tea, from which most of teas on the market are made, has similar antioxidant properties. Tea leaves are allowed to oxidize in black tea, which reduces the potency of the polyphenols.

Green tea also contains a small amount of caffeine, which in modest amounts can improve cognition. But be careful. Many people use caffeine as a substitute for getting enough sleep. If you run on caffeine, you could eventually end up developing adrenal exhaustion, which can lead to chronic fatigue!

Green tea has about 20 to 50 milligrams of caffeine per cup, compared to the 100 to 150 milligrams of caffeine per cup found in coffee. Coke, Mountain Dew, Dr. Pepper and other soft drinks have about 50 to 60 milligrams of caffeine.

Drink two to three cups of green tea per day. But don't drink it in the evenings since the caffeine in it may interfere with your ability to sleep.

DHEA

DHEA is the most abundant steroid hormone found in the bloodstream. However, there is a greater concentration of DHEA in the brain or in the neurons than in the blood. In fact, there are over six times higher concentrations of DHEA in the neurons than in the blood.

The body makes its own DHEA, and we get very little from our diet. Stress will also lower the level of DHEA as it increases the levels of cortisol, which is toxic to brain cells.

I routinely place men on DHEA. Before taking this supplement, consult your doctor and have a blood test for DHEA. In addition, get a PSA blood test and a chemistry panel, including liver function tests and a prostate exam.

Men should start by taking 50 milligrams of DHEA (or 7-keto DHEA) a day. After taking this amount for one or two months, get a second blood test for DHEA.

Men on DHEA should also take saw palmetto, at least 300 milligrams, once or twice a day to prevent enlargement of the prostate gland. Do not take DHEA supplements if you have prostate cancer.

Pregnenolone

As DHEA is known as "the mother of all steroid hormones," so pregnenolone has been called "the grandmother of all steroid hormones." The body uses pregnenolone to make testosterone, cortisone, progesterone, estrogen, aldosterone, DHEA and all other hormones in the steroid family. I usually place men on DHEA and women on pregnenolone.

Pregnenolone is not obtained from foods. Your body manufactures it from cholesterol. Large amounts of pregnenolone are produced in the brain. But those levels tend to decline as you grow older.

Many patients claim that taking this supplement improves their memory as well as their mood. I normally recommend 50–100 milligrams of pregnenolone a day. However, again, you should consult your physician prior to taking this. Both pregnenolone and DHEA may be purchased at a health food store.

This may seem like a long list of supplements! Here's what I recommend.

- If you have mild memory loss, take ginkgo and/or phosphatidyl serine.

- For moderate memory loss, add antioxidants, DHEA and choline.

- For severe memory loss, add the other supplements mentioned above.

Multivitamin Supplement

To round out your list of memory-enhancing supplements, be sure to take daily a comprehensive multivitamin/multimineral supplement that contains adequate levels of folic acid, B_6 and B_{12}. These vitamins are essential in preventing memory loss and Alzheimer's disease, and can be found in Divine Health Multivitamin.

Don't Forget Water!

It's important to drink at least two quarts of filtered

or distilled water a day. Adequate water will help detoxify your body and will help supply essential nutrients to the cells. Your brain needs plenty of water every day.

Conclusion

It takes wisdom to understand what your body needs and what it may be lacking. It also takes God's special grace to apply that wisdom to your own life. It might feel overwhelming if you didn't truly know that God loves you deeply and wants you healthy and whole, not struggling with memory loss. Like a loving father He has supplied every need you have, even in this modern world of traffic jams, deadlines and nutrient-depleted foods.

His wonderful Word assures us that He has thought about and provided for our every need. The Bible says, "And my God shall supply all your needs according to His riches in glory in Christ Jesus" (Phil. 4:19, NAS).

You can trust Him to provide for your care!

A BIBLE CURE PRAYER
FOR YOU

Dear Lord, thank You for meeting my every need. You know what vitamins, minerals, nutrients and chemicals that my body needs. You also know the exact measure of everything my brain and body may be lacking. Your Word says that even the hairs on my head are all numbered. I pray that You lead me to the supplements I need to restore any memory loss or to prevent any future memory loss. With all of my heart I thank You for Your tender loving care! In Jesus' name, amen.

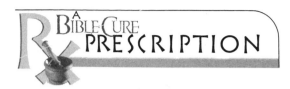

A BIBLE CURE
PRESCRIPTION

List the memory-enhancing supplements you plan to take and their dosages.

_____

_____

_____

What symptoms of memory loss have you experienced?

_____

_____

_____

Write a prayer thanking God for His provision and wisdom for your life.

_____

_____

_____

_____

Chapter 4

Exercise
for Intelligence

A healthy, well-functioning mind is a great gift from your Creator. The Bible says, "Every good gift and every perfect gift is from above" (James 1:17, NKJV). If someone gave you an expensive Rolex watch, would you wear it while gardening or treat it carelessly? Of course not! You would care for it and treasure it because of its great value. Well, the healthy, well-functioning mind that God gave you is a much more powerful gift. And you are the steward in charge of its care!

To properly care for the wonderful gift of your healthy functioning mind, you must exercise your brain. Many people do sit-ups, push-ups, jog, bicycle and walk to keep their body in top shape, but they neglect to apply the same wisdom to their minds. Let me explain.

Exercises for Brainpower

It's never too late to learn. Learning new information, regardless if you are seven or seventy years old, will cause your brain to form new dendrite connections.

But as we grow older our minds become full of trivial details. So, it's important to purge our brains of trivial details that tend to clutter our minds. We can do this by daily memorizing and meditating upon God's wonderful Word.

Write on a note card a scripture that you choose to commit to memory. Pull out the card throughout your day, reading it aloud at least three times a day or until you can repeat it without looking at it.

> *I will give you back your health and heal your wounds, says the* LORD.
> —JEREMIAH 30:17

On the following day, make a new scripture card, but don't begin memorizing it until you have read the previous day's card aloud. Add scripture upon scripture every day, starting with a complete review of all the verses in your collection.

Scripture is power-packed with the life of God, and it has an incredible effect upon the workings of your mind. The Bible says, "For the word of

God is full of living power. It is sharper than the sharpest knife, cutting deep into our innermost thoughts and desires" (Heb. 4:12).

If your mind is not cluttered up with daily insignificant details, you will be able to focus and concentrate on priority issues. A common daily activity that robs us of keen mental functioning is watching too much television. Most people watch more than four hours of TV a day, which is way too much. Why? Many television programs allow your brain to be passive, not active, and provide limited stimulation for the brain.

Researchers have found that watching excessive TV is especially harmful to children's development of spatial intelligence, which is right-brain activity. Watching TV actually causes a gradual decline in cognitive skills in many people.[1]

A BIBLE CURE HEALTH TIP

Instead of watching so much television, many brain-stimulating activities are available for leisure time. The following activities will exercise your brain:

- Reading
- Playing chess, checkers or board games
- Playing word games such as Scrabble

- Writing
- Getting involved in hobbies
- Conversing with your spouse or friends about the Bible, politics, etc.
- Reading and writing letters
- Studying the Word of God
- Listening to teaching tapes

Some television shows actually help to improve your memory. These include:

- *Jeopardy!* and other quiz shows
- Documentaries
- The Discovery Channel
- The Learning Channel

By simply turning off the TV and engaging in mental exercises, you will protect your brain, and you will stimulate new dendrite connections, thus improving your memory and preventing age-associated memory impairment.

Physical
Exercise Is Important, Too!

Not only is it important to keep using and exercising your memory and your brain, but it is also important to maintain a healthy brain through physical exercise. Physical exercise helps to reduce stress, therefore reducing cortisol levels. As mentioned earlier, high cortisol levels can be devastating to healthy brain functioning.

When you keep moving, your body will produce high amounts of vital substances that support and rescue damaged neurons from cell death. These substances are called nerve growth factors (NGF) and brain-derived neurotrophic factors (BDNF). They also help to increase the production of neurotransmitters, especially acetylcholine and dopamine.

Exercise increases oxygen and glucose to the brain and helps to remove metabolic waste from the neurons of the brain. It helps increase the production of norepinephrine and dopamine, which are neurotransmitters that give you a sense of well-being.

Since the brain uses about 25 percent of your total blood oxygen, it's easy to see how exercising to increase the flow of oxygen to the brain is one of the easiest ways of improving your memory.

Getting Started

You needn't rush out and purchase a membership to an expensive health club. You can get all the memory-building exercise you need at home. Why not consider starting a daily walking program? Brisk walking is an excellent way to improve circulation and oxygenate the blood.

Brisk Walking for Brain Power

Begin walking briskly about three to four times a week for at least twenty minutes. Walk at a pace that is comfortable for you, but walk briskly enough that you cannot sing.

You can even purchase a heart rate monitor that straps around your chest at a local sporting goods store to calculate your heart rate.

A BIBLE CURE HEALTH TIP

Your Predicted Heart Rate

To calculate your predicted heart rate, follow the formula below:

220 minus [your age] = _____
x .65 = _____ x .80 = _____

To calculate your target heart zone, follow the formula below:

220 minus [your age] = _____
x .65 = _____
[This is your minimum.]

220 minus [your age] = _____
x .80 = _____
[This is your maximum.]

This example may help: To calculate the target heart zone for a 40-year-old man, subtract the age (40) from 220 (220- 40=180). Multiply 180 by .65, which equals 117. Then multiply 180 by .80, which equals 144. A 40-year-old man's target heart rate zone is 117–144 beats per minute.

Once you have determined your desired heart rate range, write down your actual heart rate after each walking session or other exercise.

Choose an activity that you truly enjoy. Brisk walking is only one suggestion. You may decide to begin ballroom dancing lessons or backpacking. What about tennis? Or cycling? If you've never gotten involved in a regular physical activity, why not make a commitment to begin this week. Before long you may notice that you're having fewer and fewer "senior moments!"

Keeping Your Edge

If you are like so many of us, wondering if you are beginning to lose your mental edge and where it's all going to end up, stop worrying. Memory loss is common, and many people are experiencing it. Chances are, you may be experiencing a degree of memory loss along with them. But you don't have to go on stumbling for names when you introduce your friends or having to look up phone numbers that you used to recall in an instant.

Lifestyle changes are not difficult to make, even if you haven't exercised for years. I guarantee you that once you get started on an exercise program you'll begin to feel great right away. Ask God for His grace to help you to be faithful. You'll be delighted to discover how faithful and available He is to hear and answer you. Why not let me pray a prayer with you right now to ask for His help?

A Bible Cure Prayer
FOR YOU

Dear God, thank You for the gift of a well-functioning brain. I give You all my fears and concerns about memory loss. I thank You that You have provided wisdom, knowledge and help for me to live life to its fullest, free from the embarrassment and fear of memory loss. I thank You that it's Your desire for me to have a quick and keen mind throughout all my years. Please give me the grace to begin an exercise program, and help me to maintain it regularly. I thank You that You care about me deeply, that You have counted every hair upon my head and that You are truly and genuinely concerned about everything in my life. Help me to be a good steward of the incredible gift of health that You've given to me. In Jesus' wonderful name, amen.

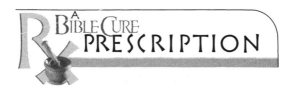

Circle the mind-enhancing exercises that you are willing to get started on right away.

memorizing scripture cards
working word puzzles
playing board games, chess or checkers
studying the Word of God
reading
getting involved with a hobby

What activities do you presently engage in that are stimulating exercises for your brain?

_____

_____

Has reading this chapter on exercising your mind influenced the television programs you plan to watch?

_____

_____

Chapter 5

Faith for a Sound Mind

G od has promised you soundness of mind:
"God has not given us a spirit of fear, but of
power and of love and of a sound mind" (2 Tim.
1:7, NKJV). Don't be frightened or discouraged by
memory loss. Through faith in God you can find
healing and help. There is nothing He cannot or
will not cure. The Bible says:

> Bless the Lord, O my soul…who heals all
> your diseases.
>
> —PSALM 103:2–3, NAS

Notice that the Bible says that God heals *all*
your diseases—He doesn't stop sending His
healing power right before He gets to memory
loss. So, have faith in God—in His love for you, in
His goodness toward you and in His desire to heal
and restore you. Faith is the final key in your

Bible cure to memory loss.

Seeing Through the Eyes of Faith

It's faith that gives us the ability to see beyond
our present circumstances into the realm of
God's perfect will for our lives. As our hearts
reach toward God's desires, the Holy Spirit
comes alongside us to help us obtain them. His
wonderful presence fills us with peace and inner
assurance that as we reach toward God, He is
also reaching back toward us.

Here are some powerful instructions about
finding God's peace:

> Don't worry about anything; instead,
> pray about everything. Tell God what you
> need, and thank him for all he has done.
> If you do this, you will experience God's
> peace, which is far more wonderful than
> the human mind can understand. His
> peace will guard your hearts and minds
> as you live in Christ Jesus.
>
> —Philippians 4:6–7

Why is peace so important? When it comes to
memory loss, stress can rob you of an accurately
functioning mind. Let's take a look.

Stress and Memory Loss

One hundred fifty years ago as settlers crossed the U.S. encountering wild animals, Indians, gunfights and natural disasters, the body's normal stress response alarm was critical for survival.

But the stress of our modern lifestyles is very different than that of our ancestors. Some modern stressors include heavy traffic, deadlines, office politics, demanding bosses, bureaucratic red tape, balancing cooking and cleaning with shuttling children to multiple activities, making ends meet financially, marital stresses, teenagers at home.

Our lifestyles create psychological stress that causes the same alarm reactions in our bodies as our ancestors experienced when their lives were threatened by wild animals or Indians. But there is one major difference. Our ancestors encountered stressful situations occasionally, but our stressors bombard us continually every day.

Our lifestyles cause high-energy chemicals to rush through our bodies hundreds of times a day, signaling our bodies to fight or flee. But we don't need to fight or flee, so we just sit and stew in our own juices. The result is ulcers, anxiety, heart problems, high blood pressure, panic attacks, tension headaches, irritable bowel syndrome and many stress-related diseases.

Three Stages of Stress

God placed the stress response in us as a mechanism of survival. Similar to shifting into passing gear on your car to accelerate and pass another vehicle, your body "shifts" into three different stages to deal with stress.

Stage 1

The first stage is the alarm stage, called *flight or fight,* when you first encounter stress. Here your mind signals your body that it is being threatened, so it begins to arm the body for possible conflict.

Your body releases adrenaline and small amounts of cortisol to begin to prepare itself for physical action. During stage 1 there is a short release of adrenaline and cortisol, and it is turned off. In stage 2 adrenaline and cortisol are continually elevated, similar to your car's accelerator being stuck.

Adrenaline races through your body, your heart beats faster and stronger, and blood rushes to your muscles and away from the stomach. Blood sugar rises, and fats are released into the bloodstream for energy. Other chemicals are also released to make the blood clot faster.

Stage 2

The second stage of stress is *resistance*. Here your body and mind try to recognize what the threat is and activate the appropriate response.

These stress chemicals are actually stimulated by a very small structure in your brain called the hypothalamus. If the stress is intense enough, as when you are in a serious car accident, for instance, or if the stress is long term, your hypothalamus sends a signal for your body to continually release these powerful chemicals. They include adrenaline and cortisol.

Although some cortisol is released during the early stages of stress, cortisol is seen as the hormone for long-term stress.

Stage 3

The third stage of the stress response is *exhaustion*. Here all of the organs that have been on heightened alert to help the body defend itself against a danger finally become exhausted.

At this stage the adrenal cortex becomes enlarged, and the spleen, lymph nodes, thymus and immune system shrink. Your entire immune system may become depleted. Your sex hormones decline, your blood pressure increases, your stomach produces excess acid, and you usually experience memory loss.

At the exhaustion phase, the cortisol levels are generally decreased. Despite feeling very tired and exhausted, you cannot sleep well. This stage of exhaustion is called the "general adaptation syndrome," and it usually accompanies a feeling that you have lost control over your life.

People with the general adaptation syndrome experience feelings of failure, being trapped and self-doubt. Many individuals at this point of stress become seriously ill.

> *He forgives all my sins and heals all my diseases.*
> —Psalms 103:3

Burnout of Chronic Stress

Over time, your mind simply burns out. The elevated cortisol levels created by chronic stress cause memory loss, eventually killing brain cells. Cortisol disrupts the function of neurotransmitters and robs the brain of glucose, which is its only energy source.

Chronic stress can also lead to depression, anxiety and chronic fatigue.

Feeling a Loss of Control

Feeling a loss of control increases stress and dramatically increases cortisol levels over the long term. The stressful lifestyle and thought patterns of learned helplessness can also result in a significant degree of memory loss.

You can develop pessimistic attitudes following various disappointments such as the loss of a job or the death of a loved one. Pessimistic attitudes can also be the result of negative belief systems stemming from childhood traumas. Such belief systems cause individuals to feel out of control when they really are not. Traumatized children grow up, but they can never seem to overcome their negative childhood experiences. As adults they may subconsciously re-create similar events in an attempt to correct those situations. For example, a woman who was abused as a child marries a man who physically abuses her. She does this unconsciously seeking to resolve her childhood conflict.

If you suffer from pessimistic attitudes and feelings of learned helplessness, the best answer is a personal relationship with Jesus Christ. Not only is God a healer of your body, but He will heal your wounded soul as well. You can revisit those negative beliefs and hurtful memories in prayer and find inner peace through God's love and forgiveness. The Holy Spirit is your comforter and teacher, and He will walk you through your painful memories and minister healing to you.

It is also critically important to forgive anyone who has wronged you and to release feelings of unforgiveness, bitterness, guilt, shame, envy and jealousy since these will also lead to a negative belief system, which will increase your stress.

Looking Up for Healing

The Word of God is powerful, for it contains the very thoughts, wisdom and understanding of God Himself. By quietly meditating upon God's Word daily, you will begin to see a transformation take place in your mind and heart.

If you hear God's Word and obey what it says, faith will rise up in you to believe for your healing. Let me encourage you to find a quiet place for daily meditation of God's Word with prayer. Through meditating upon God's Word and prayer, you will find the power of a sound mind!

A BIBLE CURE PRAYER
FOR YOU

Dear God, I thank You that You have blessed my life with a healthy functioning mind as a wonderful gift. I give You any old unresolved traumas, hurts, wounds and any other unfinished business in my soul that may be affecting my life through memory loss and other self-defeating behaviors. I choose to forgive anyone in my past or present circumstances who has hurt me. I repent for any resentment or deeply seated anger that I've harbored against anyone, including You.

Lord, I also give You my lifestyle and ask You to be a haven of peace in a stressful world. Let me know You better, and let me feel the peace of Your presence resting upon my life continually.

Thank You for filling my mind with hope and faith, and thank You for the power of a sound mind! In Jesus' name, amen.

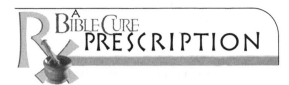

A BIBLE CURE PRESCRIPTION

Make a list of the stressors in your own life.

_____

_____

_____

Describe the symptoms of your own stress.

_____

_____

_____

Are you at stage 1, stage 2 or stage 3?

_____

List the names of everyone you choose to forgive.

_____

_____

_____

A Personal Note

From Don and Mary Colbert

God desires to heal you of disease. His Word is full of promises that confirm His love for you and His desire to give you His abundant life. His desire includes more than physical health for you; He wants to make you whole in your mind and spirit as well through a personal relationship with His Son, Jesus Christ.

If you haven't met my best friend, Jesus, I would like to take this opportunity to introduce Him to you. It is very simple.

If you are ready to let Him come into your heart and become your best friend, just bow your head and sincerely pray this prayer from your heart:

Lord Jesus, I want to know You as my Savior and Lord. I believe You are the Son of God and that You died for my sins. I also believe You were raised from the dead and now sit at the right hand of the Father praying for me. I ask You to forgive me for my sins and change my heart so that I can

be Your child and live with You eternally.
Thank You for Your peace. Help me to
walk with You so that I can begin to know
You as my best friend and my Lord. Amen.

If you have prayed this prayer, we rejoice with you in your decision and your new relationship with Jesus. Please contact us at pray4me@charismamedia.com so that we can send you some materials that will help you become established in your relationship with the Lord. You have just made the most important decision of your life. We look forward to hearing from you.

Notes

CHAPTER 1
WISDOM FOR THE WISE

1. Adapted from Dharma Khalsa, *Brain Longevity* (New York: Warner Books, Inc., 1997).
2. W. D. Heiss et al., "Activation of PET as an instrument to determine therapeutic efficacy in Alzheimer's disease," *Annals NY Acad Sci* 695 (1993): 327–331.

CHAPTER 2
FOOD FOR THOUGHT

1. For more information on how to keep your blood sugar constant, refer to my booklets *The Bible Cure for Diabetes* and *The Bible Cure for Weight Loss and Muscle Gain*.

CHAPTER 3
SUPPLEMENTS FOR BRAINPOWER

1. J. A. Joseph et al., "Oxidative stress and age-related neuronal deficits," *Molecular and Chemical Neuropathology* 28 (1996): 35–40.
2. Lester Packer, *The Antioxidant Miracle* (New York: John Wiley and Sons, Inc., 1999).
3. "Alzheimer's and Vitamin E," *New England Journal of Medicine* (April 1997).
4. Steven Bratman and David Kroll, *Natural Health Bible* (n.p.: Prima Health, 1999).
5. Pierre L. LeBars et al., "Double-blind randomized

trial of an extract of ginkgo biloba for dementia," *Journal of the American Medical Association* 278(16), (1997): 1327–1332.

6. Ibid.

7. Khalsa, *Brain Longevity*.

8. Thomas H. Crook and Brenda Adderly, *The Memory Cure* (New York: Pocket Books, 1998).

9. Bratman and Kroll, *Natural Health Bible*.

10. Frank B. Hu et al., "A prospective of cardiovascular disease in men and women," *Journal of the American Medical Association* 281(15), (1999): 1387–1394.

CHAPTER 4

EXERCISE FOR INTELLIGENCE

1. Khalsa, *Brain Longevity*.

Don Colbert, M.D., was born in Tupelo, Mississippi. He attended Oral Roberts School of Medicine in Tulsa, Oklahoma, where he received a bachelor of science degree in biology in addition to his degree in medicine. Dr. Colbert completed his internship and residency with Florida Hospital in Orlando, Florida. He is board certified in family practice and has received extensive training in nutritional medicine.

If you would like more information about natural and divine healing, or information about ***Divine Health Nutritional Products***®, you may contact Dr. Colbert at:

DR. DON COLBERT

1908 Boothe Circle
Longwood, FL 32750
Telephone: 407-331-7007
(For ordering products only)

Dr. Colbert's website is www.drcolbert.com.

Disclaimer: Dr. Colbert and the staff of Divine Health Wellness Center are prohibited from addressing a patient's medical condition by phone, facsimile or e-mail. Please refer questions related to your medical condition to your own primary care physician.

Announcing

Powerful new Divine Health products to help you live in the wonderful joy of God's divine health for you!

Divine Health™ Ginkgo Biloba

God's provision and grace extend to every area of your life, even memory loss. Ginkgo biloba is one of the most important supplements for rejuvenating memory. This powerful supplement enhances blood flow and oxygen to the brain, and it is a powerful antioxidant. Ginkgo biloba is one of the most researched botanical extracts in the world. It is used to enhance brain activity and may improve both cerebral and peripheral circulation. Divine Health Gingko Biloba is organically grown in Japan, and solvents are prohibited from being used in the extraction process. Each capsule contains 120 mg. of Ginkgo biloba leaf extract.

*Divine Health™ Proteolytic Enzymes may also be beneficial.

Pick up these great Bible Cure books by Don Colbert, MD: